MTHFR  al

A Health Journal to Optimize Genetics

Sherlock Health

substitute to seeing an actual doctor. It should be used as an educational guide to deepen your understanding of health and treatment success.

Introduction

Are you searching for answers to your MTHFR, genetic, and other health questions? The MTHFR Mutation Journal can help. Have you ever tried to improve some health symptom or problem by taking a vitamin, a supplement, or making a diet change only to have unclear results? Have you ever felt that your health was being compromised by something but just cannot put your finger on it? Maybe it is eating certain foods, some environmental trigger, or psychological factors? With MTHFR Mutation Journal you can turn those vague diet, vitamin, and supplement experiments into clear results.

This health journal is specific for those with MTHFR and other genetic mutations. It is for the self-experimenter, biohacker, and curious person who really wants to understand how different things are influencing their health. Let's face it, your genetic factors are hard enough to keep track of. You don't live in a bubble and there are a lot of confounding factors influencing your health from one day to the next like; travel, diet changes, mental factors, emotional influences, family changes, and more. Get clarity on what is and what is not influencing your genetics and health with MTHFR Mutation Journal

MTHFR Mutation Journal will help you make connections about what is influencing your health. Many times the reason you struggle is from uncertainty and feeling overwhelmed. Uncertainty on what is and is not working. Uncertainty about how your diet is affecting you, uncertainty about your sleep schedule, your digestion, and many things you have not even considered.

You can't change your genetics but through continually asking yourself questions, like the ones in this journal, you can make them work better. Journaling and looking at these questions will help you pay closer attention. This attention will bring a deeper understanding of the health factors you can control. This creates clarity. With this clarity, the solutions will be much easier to see. This health journal and notebook was developed to help train your mind to look for and find answers to your genetic health issues. Think of it as a way to help yourself and your doctor better understand how different things are influencing your health. It will give you more certainty about how medicines, vitamins, supplements or diets are or are not helping you. Perhaps, more importantly, it can be used to further refine what the cause of your health issues are.

The Questions

General and Environmental Questions

- How do you respond in different weather environments?
    - o Why do you think that is?
- Do certain seasons or weather patterns seem to bring on health ailments?
    - o Why?
- How do you feel at work versus home?
- How does stress affect your symptoms?
- Is there anything different about your symptoms when you are on vacation that suggests your home is causing your symptoms?
- Any problems with elevation?
- When you stay in different homes or go on vacation to certain areas do you have any changes in your health status?
- What do environmental toxins do to your health in the immediate and long term?
- How much toxins are you exposed to?
    - o What can you do to protect yourself?
- Do you use chemicals to clean with in your home?
- Do you use chemicals on your clothes?

Diet Questions

- What foods do you feel best with?
    - o Why?
- How many different types of diets are there?
- What are some categories of foods that can cause health issues?
- Is there a way to look at the foods that impact you as a category?
- Are there any foods that many people have problems with?
- How much water do you drink?
- How much protein should you eat per day?
    - o Why?
- How much protein do you consume?
- Do you eat high, moderate, or low carb diet?
    - o How do you know?
- What is the role of food on your immune system?
- How did your last meal affect your immune system?
- Do you know why organic is better for you?
    - o When do you choose organic foods over conventional?
- How often do you eat breads and pasta made of gluten?
    - o How many should you have?

- How many servings of sugary snacks do you have daily?
  - o How much is too much?
- Eating later in the day is more likely to cause weight gain than eating early
- How much plain water do you drink each day?
  - o How much should you drink?

Digestive Questions

- How often do you have a bowel movement?
- How does your digestion change from one day to the next?
- What color are your stools?
- Do they have odor?
    - o If so what does it smell like?
- Do your stools sink or float?
    - o Why does this matter?
- Do you know what an optimal stool looks like
    - o How do you know?
- How do we distinguish good bacteria from bad bacteria?
- What do you do to promote good bacteria verses bad bacteria?
- How much gas is normal to have in one day
    - o How does this compare to you?
- You can improve your digestion after a meal by lying on your right, lying on back, or lying on left?
- Certain foods cause gas, diarrhea, or heartburn.
    - o Those foods are….
- What are some signs of poor skin health?
- Does diet affect your skin?

Mental and Mood Questions

- How do you know when your emotions are balanced?
- Have you been frustrated in the last couple days?
    - o What caused this frustration?
- Are there emotions that you feel more of during certain times of the year, or month?
- How do you manage your stress?
    - o Are there certain activities or exercises that help you?
- Are there ways to manage your emotions?
- How do you respond to different social settings?
    - o Why do you think that is?
- Do you worry about what might happen in the future?
    - o Where does this come from?
- When you feel sad what role do other people play in this?
    - o How much control do you have?
- Does exercise change your mental and emotional health?
- Do you go to sleep without trouble?
    - o How long does it take you to fall asleep?

- When you wake in the am are you well rested or groggy?
    - o Does this suggest anything?
- Do you feel tired during the day at certain points?
- Where does the energy in your body come from?
    - o How does your body make it?

MTHFR and Methylation Questions

- What does the MTHFR enzyme do for your body?
- How do you think this mutation has affected your health?
  - When did it start?
- What doe the overall methylation process do for your body?
- What are non-genetic factors that affect methylation?
- How do you know if you are getting enough or too much methylation?
- When you take methylfolate do you feel better, worse or the same?
  - In what way?
- Does methylfolate give you any headaches or worsen your headaches?
- With methylfolate do you feel more anxious and worried or excited and free?
- Does methylfolate make your body have a heavy feeling?
- Any increase in joint aches or body pains?
- Do you have new or continuing numbness or tingling?

- What are methyl donors?
    - o Should you take these?
- Are there dietary things that can help or hurt your methylation?
    - o Have you experimented to find the empirical value of these?
- How do you know if you are getting too much or too little methylfolate or other methylation sport?

Immune Questions

- How often do you get sick?
    - o Does this seem to be more, less or equal to those around you?
- What process brings on allergic reactions in your body?
- Are there things that trigger your allergies?
    - o Is there a time when it is worse?
- Do you get urinary tract infections very often?
- Are you more vulnerable to illness in summer or winter?
- Where does inflammation in your body come from?
- Do you have inflammation in your body?
    - o How would you know?

Physical Health Questions

- How many push ups can you do?
    - o How many do you think you should be able to do?
- How long would it take you to run a mile?
    - o Should you be able to run a mile at your age?
- Do you find it difficult to loose weight?
    - o Why do you think that is?
- What kind of relationship do you have with your food?
- What is your ideal weight?

Journal Pages

Made in United States
North Haven, CT
17 June 2023

37868208R00071